# GROW YOUR HAIR, CHANGE YOUR LIFE

## THE BLACK WOMEN'S GUIDE TO GROWING AND MAINTAINING LONG, HEALTHY, SHINY HAIR

### LERI SMITH

Dedicated to my son, Ellis, who inspires me to grow every day.

"When we accept things about ourselves, including our hair, and love those things about ourselves, true growth will happen!"

- Leri Smith, Author

GROW YOUR HAIR, CHANGE YOUR LIFE

# TABLE OF CONTENTS

# Introduction
## Grow Your Hair - Grow Yourself!

As a young black woman, I always believed that I could not grow my hair long. I had been led to believe that black women have kinky, unmanageable hair. Hair that will never be flowing, shiny tresses like other races of women!

I never liked this philosophy and decided, against all odds, that I was going to grow my hair - one way or another! I for one, was not going to become a hostage to my hair! After all, when was the last time hair ran the show?

I was determined to go forward with a total attitude of success! I was going to let my hair know who's boss!

With this new mindset, I set out on my quest - Do or Die - To Grow My Hair! Through determination and my new found "Do Not Take No For An Answer" - My Hair Grew! Yes! Long - Flowing Tresses of Hair!

Now, you might well ask, what has hair got to do with it? Let me tell you what happened to me when I discovered I could grow my hair. Once I changed my belief regarding the capabilities of my hair, I was able to discover what I, as a person, am capable of changing and doing within myself. By exploring the myth that Black women cannot grow long hair, I was able to explore other myths that have clung to me most of my life. I started examining my own beliefs about money, race and beauty!

When we overlook or avoid issues of our physical being - i.e. our hair, we often will do the same with our spiritual self as well. When we accept things about ourselves, including our hair, and love those things about ourselves, true growth will happen!

www.ShareHairSecrets.com

Because of my quest for long hair, I discovered a hidden quest within myself. Through nurturing and love, anything is possible including the acceptance of ourselves in our own eyes.

This journey has inspired me to write an eBook 50 Hair Do's and Dont's and now this book, Grow Your Hair, Change Your Life. What you Don't do for your hair is just as important as what you Do for your hair. What you *don't* do for yourself, as well as what you *do* for yourself, will have a large impact on your life and your successes!  Cure of one's own spirit comes from within. Healthy hair also comes from within. What you eat, what you drink, relief from stress, appropriate rest; all these things play a big part in healthy hair and a healthy outlook. I will show you how to have healthy, long, flowing hair. Come along with me on an inspirational journey into body and mind.

Knowledge brings order and harmony to every aspect of our lives. The recognition of how everything in our lives is connected, comes from a positive attitude. Great things happen in our minds, bodies, and yes, our hair, when we learn to grow.

## Hair Peace

Having long, healthy, shiny hair is about how you take care of it. What you do to it and what you don't do. This book is guide to show you a step-by-step method for growing and maintaining long healthy, shiny hair. Too many of us do not have the slightest idea of how to grow and maintain shiny healthy hair. Instead, we like to go for the quick fix of extensions, wigs and relaxers, but the only thing we get quickly is breakage.

What many of us fail to realize is that "cure" comes from within. Our attitudes and beliefs,  as well as our good health habits, determine our hair length. Many of us believe that Black woman simply do not grow hair. For any of us who have ever tried to color, relax or cover gray, know that our hair grows faster than we want it to, sometimes. So why is it that so many of us do not have long hair? Most of us learned at an early age, while our moms or grandmothers were yanking and pulling on our little kinks, that our hair was bad, something to fight with, something to hate. So we've learned to put off doing it. Or have someone else deal with it. But you have to love your own hair and be willing to play with it in order for it to grow.

1. **Be gentle with your hair!** Use only a wide toothed comb.

2. **Nurture your hair daily** with olive oil and coconut oil.

3. **Protect your hair,** always wrap it or roll it at night.

4. **Treat your hair right;** apply a hair mask and hot oil treatment every month.

5. **Stimulate your scalp** by massaging it for a few minutes each day.

What many of us don't realize is that once we come to peace with our hair, it will grow. Once we stop trying to change it or add to it, it will grow. Anything that grows must be nurtured and loved. Think about a houseplant. Would you add chemicals or color to it and still expect it to grow? Just like a plant, you must nurture your hair and care for it everyday. What you don't do to your hair is often just as important or more important than what you do to your hair.

All individuals must take an active role in the growing and upkeep of their hair's health. The more we learn about nutrition, and proper maintenance the better prepared we will be to take an active role.

Attitude is also an important factor in the process of health and maintenance of your hair. We must have a positive state of mind in order to bring harmony to every aspect of our lives. The recognition of how everything in our lives is connected will help us to grow in mind, body, spirit and of course hair.

# .1.

## THE TRUTH ABOUT OUR HAIR

There is no chemical difference in the makeup of African-American hair in comparison with any other hair type. It has a cuticle (the outer layer), a cortex (the middle layer, composed primarily of keratin and moisture, plus melanin, which gives our hair its color), and a medulla (the center of the hair shaft).

Black hair textures can vary from fine to medium to coarse; its curl pattern from straight to softly wavy to excessively tight; its colors from blonde to red, to all sorts of browns, to black.

All hair grows ½ inch a month. Although there is a genetically predetermined hair cycle from 2 years to 7 years, even if you are on the two-year cycle your hair could be 12 inches long if you took proper care of it.

Black hair is usually coarser in texture, tighter in curl pattern, more naturally delicate, and more vulnerable to damage from chemical treatments.

The average head has 10,000 strands of hair that grow about ½ inch per month.

Longer hair is older and has gone through lots of washing, combing, brushing, heat styling, and chemicals.

Hair is dead once it leaves your scalp. Although it is very strong, it has no way of healing itself once it is damaged.

# Hair Growth Myths

**MYTH #1: Braids make your hair grow.**

Truth:  When your hair is braided, you are able to see the new growth that would occur whether or not your hair is braided. Healthy hair grows ½ inch per month.

**Myth #2:  Trimming makes your hair grow.**

Truth:  Trimming your hair stops split ends from traveling up the hair shaft, which stops breakage, but growth occurs from your scalp.

**Myth #3: Relaxers make your hair grow.**

Truth: Relaxers make your hair appear longer because they straighten your natural curls, but can be very damaging.

**Myth #4: Greasing your scalp makes your hair grow.**

Truth: Greasing you scalp clogs your hair follicles and pores on your scalp. This makes it difficult for your scalp to breathe and can make it difficult for hair growth.

**Myth #5: Natural styles make your hair grow.**

Truth:  Chemicals and heat styling are more damaging to hair, but kinky natural styles can be just as damaging if not combed properly from daily wear and tear.

Hair growth occurs with a good diet and healthy maintenance. Taking vitamins, drinking water, eating nutritious foods and trimming split ends.

# .2.

## Choosing Products

### Shampoo

Our hair is generally drier than most hair types, so I recommend always using a moisturizing shampoo and conditioner. Never use a shampoo designed for oily hair. They contain deep cleansing properties designed to remove oils and build-up, but they are extremely harsh on our hair. They completely strip our hair of needed natural oils.

Do not use shampoos with sulfates, silicones, glycols. When choosing shampoo, choose a shampoo without Sodium Lauryl Sulfate, which is a foaming agent that is not good for your hair and very bad for your health in large quantities. Sodium Laureth Sulfate is a much better choice when choosing a shampoo. It is very important to read the ingredients. They take moisture out of black hair, cause dryness, brittleness and can create scalp conditions.

Instead, choose only moisturizing shampoos. They are designed for dry hair.

### Conditioners

Always use a moisturizing conditioner. When choosing a conditioner, notice how your hair responds. If it tightens and tangles, do not use it. If your hair loosens and combs through easily, then you have found a good conditioner.

It is always good to have 2 – 3 different shampoos and conditioners, so that you can switch up every couple of weeks. Change the brand of conditioner you use every few months, since hair can become immune to a specific formula's effects, and build-up can occur.

It is not important to use a shampoo and conditioner by the same company. Some companies make better shampoos, others make better conditioners.

## LEAVE-IN PRODUCTS

Leave-in products are very important because they protect your hair from heat and styling damage. Most leave-in products protect your hair from dryness and brittleness that is caused by thermal styling. They also help prevent breaking and split ends by adding moisture to your hair.

Leave-in products are designed to moisturize, repair dry damaged hair, add shine, control frizz, detangle your hair, prevent split ends, stop hair breakage, enhance natural body, and act as a thermal protector.

Do not use heavy creams, lotions, and greases. Avoid mineral oil or petroleum-based products.

## WIDE-TOOTH COMB

The number one way to lose hair is using the wrong comb. We all have to comb our hair; unless we have locks or a very short hair style. The most natural way to separate tangles is with our fingers, and a wide-toothed comb emulates this.

The teeth on your comb are too small if you see more than a few hairs in your comb everyday. A wide-toothed comb is good for the fine hair as well as the kinkiest hair. It is a must for hair growth. Wash your comb with shampoo or hand soap before each use.

When choosing a wide toothed comb, it is best to choose one without seams, which can be rough on the hair. Handmade wide-tooth combs made out of cellulose acetate are best.

## CLIPS

You will need at least 4 plastic hair clips before starting your hair routine. They will assist you in keeping your hair pinned up while working in sections. You will need to keep the damp and dry hair apart. Use the plastic hair clips that open and close easily and can hold a large amount of hair. Avoid the long metal clips; they tend to rip out hair.

## BLOW DRYER

A quality blow dryer is a must if you want healthy strong hair that isn't brittle or frayed. Cheaper blow dryers use metal or plastic heating elements that dry your hair by cooking the water off of your hair.

Quality dryers use ceramic heating, usually infused with tourmaline, which is great for heat conduction and penetrates the hair shaft much more safely because the heat is gentler and safer.

Ionic blow dryers produce negatively charged ions, which causes the cuticle to remain flat. This traps in moisture. Cheaper blow dryers produce positive ions that cause the cuticle to open. This leaves the hair frizzy and damaged.

## FLAT IRON

A quality flat iron is very important for your hair's health. It is important that your flat iron has adjustable heat settings between 140°F and 200°F.

The flat iron must have ceramic plates and tourmaline technology, because they heat more evenly, are smoother on the hair, and cause less damage. The tourmaline emits negative-ions, which leave hair shiny and silky.

For shorter hair, buy a flat iron with 1/2 to 1-inch plates. For longer hair, buy a flat iron with 1-3/8 to 2 inch plates.

## SHEARS/SCISSORS

Only use a pair of hair shears. Regular scissors are not sharp enough and can cause more split ends. You can buy them at a local beauty supply.

Household scissors will damage your hair. Do not cut anything else but your hair with your shears and make sure that no one else uses them to cut anything but hair.

## HAIR WRAP

Daily maintenance is extremely important for growing your hair. Wrapping your hair every night is one of the most important steps that you will take to protect your ends.  Wrapping your hair keeps your hair healthy and prevents breakage.

Wrapping also keeps your hair straight so you will not have to touch up your hair during the week with heat styling products.

Use satin or silk scarf or bonnet to tie your hair up at night. Cotton pillowcases can be too rough on the hair and cause breakage. They can also absorb the oil from your hair.

If wrapping your hair is not possible, use a silk or satin pillowcase.

## SATIN BONNET

A satin bonnet is good to have for sleeping and for showering. Make sure that it fits snuggly around your hair and that it completely covers all of your edges.

## ROLLERS

Way before electric curling irons were invented, women rolled their hair with rollers. This is my curling preference because there is no heat used, it takes less time, it protects your ends while you sleep, and it is easy.

The bendable foam rollers are best. The plastic ones with a clip or the open ones that require bobby pins and sponge rollers often leave indentations in your hair and can be uncomfortable when you sleep.

## SHOWER CAP

You can buy a shower cap at most beauty supply stores. It is a must if you want to maintain and protects heat styled hair.

## PLASTIC CAPS

You will need plastic caps for deep conditioning treatments. They help your hair to stay moist and retain heat, which helps for penetration of the deep conditioner.

## SATIN PILLOW CASE

Wrapping your hair is highly recommended, but it is great to have a silk or satin pillowcase for those lazy nights.

# .3.

## How to Wash Your Hair

### Before You Wash

Our hair is very delicate and can be very brittle if it is too dry. It is important to apply a generous amount of Conditioner before you begin combing out your hair.

Before you wash your hair, it is important to make sure that it is combed out well. If you do not detangle your hair, the loose hairs will tangle back into your hair during washing and you will pull out more hair than necessary after washing.

### Washing Your Hair

Washing your hair once a week is best. Washing more than once a week can be drying, and washing your hair less often can cause scalp conditions. When you wash your hair once a week, you stimulate blood circulation on the scalp; you open the hair follicles, which promote hair growth. You also reduce the product build-up, dirt, and germs, which cause scalp conditions.

Going longer than one to two weeks makes your hair dry and brittle and causes breakage. Your hair needs the nourishment from water and conditioners. Your hair needs to be washed often to get rid of dirt, grime, oils and products that weigh it down. It also needs conditioner to revitalize it. Most importantly, it needs the water to hydrate it every week or two.

## ഔ 1 ര

It is important to keep your scalp clean for hair growth. If you have a flaky scalp, gently brush dandruff with a toothbrush. Exfoliate your scalp by scratching all flakes and dandruff off of your scalp.

Do not comb your hair with the small toothed-comb. It will pull your hair out.  Be gentle to your scalp, there should be no blood or pain.  For easier removal, first apply warm olive oil to your scalp; it's a great hot oil treatment, too.

# ℘ 2 ℥

Gently use a wide-toothed comb to comb your hair from the ends to the roots. Do not yank your hair or force a comb through the tangles. You will pull out healthy hair unnecessarily.

This step is important for removing all of the loose hairs out of your hair so they will not tangle back into your hair when washing. Remove any excess hair that appears on the comb before you begin combing the next section. This prevents loose hair from tangling back into your hair.

# ℘ 3 ℥

Use luke-warm to cool water to rinse your hair. Be sure that you rinse your hair for at least 30 seconds before you apply shampoo to ensure that all of your hair and scalp are saturated with water.

Do not use hot water to wash your hair. It strips away natural oils and causes your hair and scalp to be dry. The water should be as cool as you can take it, even in the winter.

# ℘ 4 ℥

When applying your shampoo, apply it directly to the scalp and let it lather into your hair. Too much shampoo can dry out your hair.

# ❧ 5 ☙

Massage your entire scalp to lift up all flakes.

# ❧ 6 ☙

Rinse your scalp thoroughly with cool water. Rinse for at least 1 – 2 minutes to ensure that all of the shampoo is gone.

# ❧ 7 ☙

Apply a quarter-sized amount of shampoo into your hair, if it lathers up quickly, you know that your hair is clean. If not, apply a little more shampoo and massage into your hair.

Never wash your hair more than twice. Washing it more than twice will dry out your hair and scalp.

# ❧ 8 ☙

Rinse your scalp thoroughly. Rinse for at least 1 – 2 minutes to ensure that all of the shampoo is gone.

# ❧ 9 ☙

Gently squeeze out all the excess water, but do not dry with a towel.

# .4.

## How to Condition Your Hair

### ‽ 1 ଔ

Choose a conditioner that is right for your hair type. Choose a quality conditioner to maintain healthy hair.

Every month use a deep conditioner on your hair and sit under a dryer or wrap it with a hot towel for 45 minutes to one hour.

### ‽ 2 ଔ

Apply a generous amount of conditioner to your hair. Start with your ends, since it is the oldest part of your hair, and work the conditioner to the top of your hair.

### ‽ 3 ଔ

Comb your hair with your wide-toothed comb while the conditioner is still in your hair. The conditioner will protect your hair from harsh pulling and it will be less tangled after you rinse your hair.

It is easier to detangle your hair while the conditioner is still in it. Your hair is weaker when it is wet, so the conditioner helps protect your hair. Remove all loose hairs from your comb as much as possible so the loose hairs do not tangle in your hair.

If you skip this step, loose hairs will re-tangle in your hair and combing it out will pull out a lot of healthy hairs. Your hair will also be more tangled and harder to deal with.

## ‮ഉ‬ 4 ‮ଓ‬

Rinse your hair thoroughly with cool water, but it is okay to leave a little bit of conditioner in your hair.

## ‮ഉ‬ 5 ‮ଓ‬

Blot your hair with a clean towel. Your hair is at its weakest when wet. When using a towel, never rub the towel on your hair. The friction can cause the hair to weaken or break. Always blot or pat the water out of your hair without rubbing or tugging your hair.

# .5.

## How to Blow Dry Your Hair

## Before You Blow Dry Your Hair

Always use a leave-in conditioner or a thermal heat protector after you wash and condition your hair, but make sure you do not use more than a quarter sized amount because it will cause build-up and possibly flake off of your hair.

## ಜಾ 1 ಲ

Apply a leave-in conditioner to your wet hair. Pay special attention to your ends, which is the part of your hair that needs the leave-in conditioner the most, since it is your oldest and most damaged hair.

Avoid putting the leave-in conditioner on your scalp. It will only cause build-up and block your hair follicles. The new hair at your roots does not need as much conditioning as your ends.

## ಜಾ 2 ಲ

It is very important to divide your hair into small manageable sections because it causes fewer tangles. Divide your hair into 4 - 6 manageable sections and braid them or clip them.

If your hair is not long enough to braid, use clips to clip your hair into manageable sections. Continue to re-braid your hair into small manageable section until you straighten it.

If you do not divide your hair into manageable sections, it will be harder to deal with and your hair will get tangles again, which means more hair will be pulled out. You want to avoid having to comb your hair too many times while it is wet.

## ℘ 3 ℘

Always detangle your hair using a wide-toothed comb. Start with the ends of your hair and work your way up to the roots. If you start from the roots down to the ends, you will cause your hair to break.

If you have the type of hair that doesn't tangle or nap up, air-drying is the best for your hair.

### BLOW DRYING YOUR HAIR

Do not blow-dry your hair more than once a week; it can be very drying and damaging to your hair.

You can use the highest setting on your blow dryer, but always keep the blow dryer moving through your hair. Never allow the blow dryer to be in one spot for more than a second or two, because it will burn your hair.

## ℘ 1 ℘

Unbraid one section; hold your hair with one hand and the hair dryer with the other so that your hair is not flying all over and tangling. Work the hair dryer form your scalp to the ends. Avoid applying too much heat to your ends. Braid that section again.

# ಲ 2 ಛ

Repeat with all the sections and re-braid each section after you dry it.

With the proper drying technique, you will be able to dry your hair and scalp in the shortest amount of time, causing less heat damage.

Hint: If your scalp feels cool, part of your hair is still wet. Move the blow dryer around your head until your scalp is completely dry.

# .6.

## How to Flat Iron Your Hair

When flat ironing your hair, it is important to begin with healthy, well-conditioned hair. Any type of heat styling can be damaging to your hair. If you hair is not already healthy, you may not get the results that you want and you will further damage your hair.

It is possible to have healthy hair that is flat ironed. I have been flat ironing my hair every week for many years and it remains healthy, but I began with healthy hair. And I only flat iron my newly washed and well-conditioned hair.

Never apply heat to dirty hair. Applying heat to hair with product build-up and dirt will only cake the dirt into your hair, which is damaging and stinky. It may be tempting to touch up your hair with the flat iron during the week, but remember, that is short-term satisfaction. Your long-term goal is long, beautiful, healthy, shiny hair.

## ഇ 1 ശ

Only flat iron dry, newly washed, well-conditioned hair.  Apply a leave-in conditioner, balm, or heat protector first.

## ഇ 2 ശ

Pre-heat your flat iron at least 5 minutes before use. Although most flat-irons have a temperature setting that goes up to 450°F, 200°F is sufficient for most of your flat iron needs.

Experiment with 200°F first, and only increase the heat if 200°F doesn't get the results that you need. Try 250°F, then 300°F, etc.

# ೫ 3 ೫

Section off your hair into 4 to 6 small, easy to manage sections. It is better to start in the back of your hair and work your way up to the top.

# ೫ 4 ೫

Part your hair into small rows about 1 inch thick. Do not press pieces wider or thicker than 1 inch at a time. It will be easier and more effective for you to straighten the entire section if you work with small sections of hair at a time. If you try to straighten too much hair at one time, it will not be as effective.

# ೫ 5 ೫

Start as close to the roots as possible. Pull the iron down in one smooth motion. Go slowly. One slow pull through is better than two or three fast ineffective ones. The less heat you put in your hair, the better.

Remember, never stop and let the iron sit in one place on your hair, it will damage your hair, and possibly burn it.

# ೫ 6 ೫

Flat iron the other sections of your hair the same way. Once the hair is straightened, do not clip, braid or tie the hair. This will cause an indentation in your hair.

# .7.

## How to Trim Your Hair

All trims do not require a trip to the salon. If you learn how to trim your own split ends, you can keep your hair looking healthy between visits. If you want a cut or a hairstyle, you should definitely go to a professional hair stylist. These recommendations are simply for the health and maintenance of your hair.

## Trim Your Hair Every 8 to 12 Weeks

Trimming your hair is essential for long hair. Split ends will continue to split if they are not trimmed.

If you are serious about having long hair, you should cut off all damaged hair. If that is too heartbreaking, trim off one inch every two months. It will help you maintain the same length since your hair grows a half an inch per month. Once all damaged hair is trimmed off, trim your hair every 8 – 12 weeks.

If you trim your hair yourself, buy very sharp hair shears. These scissors should only be used to cut hair. It is important to inform everyone in your home not to use them to cut anything else.

Only trim freshly washed, conditioned and straightened hair. Do not replace trimming your hair with split end "mending" products. They just temporarily mend the ends together.

## ℘ 1 ℘

Only use a pair of hair shears. Regular scissors are not sharp enough and can cause more split ends.

# ಸಂ 2 ಲ

When you cut your hair, always cut perpendicular. If you cut your hair at and angle or a slant, your ends won't be as strong and will split easier.

# ಸಂ 3 ಲ

When you make a cut, be sure to cut at least a 1/4 of an inch above the split end. This way you will know that you have cut off all of the dry damaged hair and to ensure that you will have a healthy end.

# ಸಂ 4 ಲ

It is always good to trim your hair in a well-lit area. A backlight or the sun is highly recommended.

## DUSTING

Dusting is a form of trimming your hair where you cut just one strand of hair at a time. Although dusting is time consuming, this method is highly recommended for those of us that are new to cutting our own hair.

# ಸಂ 1 ಲ

Take a small section of hair and twist it. You will see the ends of your hair pop up. Cut each hair individually about ¼ of an inch above the end.

Or you can just hold a small section in front of a backlight or the sun.

# ৪০ 2 ଓଃ

Grab another section of hair and repeat until you have dusted all of your hair.

# .8.

## Daily Maintenance

### Bedtime

Always cover your hair at night. You must protect your ends. This is true for natural hairstyles, presses and perms. The rubbing of your ends against your cotton pillowcase is devastating for your hair. It causes your ends to split unnecessarily, and the cotton absorbs the natural oils from your hair.

Wrapping your hair at night allows your hair to retain moisture and helps you maintain your hairstyle. When your hair is nice and neat, you will not have to touch it up with heat.

The most convenient hair wrap is a stocking cap, satin/silk bonnet or scarf.

You can also roll your hair with bendable foam rollers. Divide your hair into 4 sections. Just use 1 roller in each section to avoid curls that are too tight.

Put just a little bit of oil or moisturizer on your ends every couple of days.

Avoid, as much as possible, leaving your hair uncovered at night. If wrapping or rolling your hair is unbearable, use a satin pillowcase. This is a much better option than a cotton pillowcase, but your ends will rub against it and possibly split.

## SHOWER

Always wrap your hair in a satin bonnet. Put a plastic shower cap over your satin cap. Be sure that all of the edges of your hair are completely covered and that the shower cap is snug to prevent steam from entering into the cap and causing your hair to frizz up.

## MORNING

Your morning routine will be pretty simple if you tie your hair at night. Unwrap or unroll your hair and use your fingers to style or work through any tangles.

## A HEALTHY BODY MAKES HEALTHY HAIR

## WATER

Water is a nutrient so it is important to drink 8 glasses everyday.

## NUTRITIOUS FOODS

Having a diet rich in fruits, vegetables, whole grains, fish, and chicken will give your body the nutrients needed for healthy hair. Check out *www.SaladBS.com* for a great salad you can make 2-5 times a week, that you'll love!

## EXERCISE

Exercise promotes hair growth because it stimulates blood flow. When blood flows to the hair follicles it carries nutrients needed for hair growth. When blood flow to the hair follicles is low, it results in dull, brittle hair. Exercise also reduces stress. Stress can cause hair loss.

## VITAMINS

Drink a green powder supplement, a liquid vitamin or take a multivitamin. Hair vitamins are available. Some people swear by pre-natal vitamins.  It doesn't really matter, choose the one that best suits your life style, but choose one.

## Sleep

When we sleep, our body repairs and regenerates itself.  When we do not get enough sleep, our body does not have a chance to recharge, and this can cause hair loss.  It is recommended that we get eight hours of sleep per night.  When we don't get enough sleep, it will not only affect our hair growth, but it can also cause hair loss.

## Eliminate Unhealthy Habits

## Junk Food

Bad hair days occur when we don't get enough vitamins or protein. Bad nutrition causes hair loss. A diet low in nutrients is linked to hair loss. Reduce caffeine, alcohol, and nicotine.

## Cleansing

Cleansing your intestines is critical to attaining great health as we get older. One product that comes highly recommended is ALOE CLEANSE. You can find details about this great cleansing product at *www.ColonBS.com*. Use this product the morning after eating junk food or a heavy weekend of food or beverage consumption. Doing this will allow your body to absorb needed nutrients from the good foods you eat. Without nutrients, your hair has little chance of growing thick and full.

## Stress

Any kind of stress, whether emotional or physical, can lead to hair loss.  A condition known as telogen effluvim can cause sudden and rapid hair loss due to physical stresses like illness or childbirth.

If you have emotional or psychological stress, it can interfere with the normal growth cycle of the hair.  If you suffer from hair loss due to stress, there are many ways you can reduce stress in your life, such as rest and exercise, to help restore hair growth.

# .9.

## HAIR DON'TS

### Grease your Scalp

Greasing your scalp actually clogs your pores. This can prohibit scalp circulation and hair growth. It is, however, great to apply moisturizers to your ends.

### Soft Bristle Brush

If you must brush your hair, a boar's bristle brush is much better than those nylon or plastic ones. However, any type of brush can be too rough and rip out your hair, damage hair follicles and cause breakage. If you really want long healthy hair, throw away all hairbrushes. Use a wide-tooth comb only.

### Braids, Weaves, Wigs and Buns

Braids and buns are highly recommended to give your hair a rest from heat styling. However, you must avoid those styles that are braided too tightly. They will cause hair breakage and even permanent hair loss if your follicles are damaged. If you wear braids often, make sure you allow your hair to rest for a few weeks between braids.

Do not wear your hair just one-way. Every hairstyle has its pros and cons that put a strain on your hair. It is important to alternate between natural hairstyles, braids or weaves, and straightening your hair.

If you wear braids most of the time, take a few months off and wear your hair down. If you wear your hair down most of the time, take a few months and get braids or a weave.

Never get weave tracks glued into your hair, you will surely have hair loss when the tracks are removed. Never leave a weave or braids in your hair longer than two months.

It is nice to wear your hair in a bun, but keep it looser rather than tight. Never use hairpins or bobby pins if the little round bulbs are missing from the ends. Take your bun down at night and avoid sleeping in rubber bands and pins.

Wearing a wig all day long is not good for your hair or scalp because they need to breathe. They can also damage and break your edges due to rubbing.

## CHEMICALS

You do not need chemicals, like color, bleach, relaxers or texturizers to have long flowing hair. All chemicals are very damaging to your hair.

## RELAXERS

Advertisers promise that Natural relaxers and no-lye relaxers are better for your hair, but they are not. Any type of relaxer is damaging to your hair because they all contain chemicals. No-lye relaxers have less sodium hydroxide, but it still has damaging chemicals. You can have straight flowing healthy hair by following to techniques offered in this book.

## SWIMMING

It is best to avoid swimming because chlorine is very damaging to your hair. If you swim often, make sure you wash your hair as soon as you get out of the pool. It is best to wear braids if you swim often. The braids will allow you to wash your hair each time without having to comb it out and cause breakage. Apply conditioner to your hair before and after swimming.

Do not let the chlorine or salt water dry in your hair.  Always wash and condition it right away.

## PONYTAILS

Wear your hair down as much as possible.  If you commit to doing your hair once a week, it will always look good.

If you must wear your hair in a ponytail, do not slick your hair back with gel or anything else.  Gels contain alcohol that dries and damages your hair.  Slicking your hair back with a brush causes severe damage to your follicles and permanent hair loss.

## RUBBER BANDS

Avoid using rubber bands with the metal fasteners.  Use the elastic snag-free type instead.  They are smoother and glide off of your hair without pulling or breaking your hair.

## HEAD BANDS

Sometimes the hard plastic headbands can damage your hair.  Choose elastic or soft cloth ones.  They are gentler on your hair.

## SHARING HAIR UTENSILS

It is very important not to use other people's hair utensils.  It is unhygienic and can transmit dandruff, and other hair disorders.

Cleaning your combs and brushes with soap and water everyday will clear up any problems you have with dry scalp and dandruff because you are not constantly adding dirt and grim back to your scalp.

## DEGREASERS

Do not use dishwashing liquid or other degreasers on your hair.  It strips your hair of the essential natural oils your hair needs and dries out your hair.

If you have product build-up follow the Apple cider vinegar recipe in the back of this book to get rid of residue build-up on hair.

## PRODUCTS

Most products promise unrealistic results. Save your money on other hair care products like gel and hair growth products. Most hair growth products don't actually give the promised results and you are putting random hormones on your scalp that seeps into your bloodstream. Who knows what they will cause to grow unnaturally once they get into your body.

There is no way to grow hair instantly. Do not fall for gimmicks that promise fast hair growth.

## SPEAK UP

Do not give the responsibility of your hair growth to someone else. If you allow a hairstylist to do your hair, speak up if he/she is yanking, breaking, or burning out your hair. Once a hair has left your head, it is gone forever. When you spend time nurturing and growing your hair, only go to others that nurture your hair like you do.

# .10.

## Homemade Hair Care Recipes

### Flaky Scalp*

After you wash your hair, mix 1 cup of apple cider vinegar with a ½ cup of warm water. Pour over entire scalp, massage and let is dry. Do not rinse out.

For tougher dandruff and flaky scalp, apply undiluted apple cider vinegar directly to your scalp with a cotton ball. Leave on for 15 minutes. Rinse out and apply conditioner to cover the smell.

### To Remove Build-Up*

Add a 2 tablespoons of apple cider vinegar to 1 quart of warm water. Pour it over your hair after shampooing.

### Honey For Shine

After you wash and condition your hair, add 1 tablespoon of honey to 1 quart of warm water. Pour on your hair. Leave it in.

### Honey and Olive Oil Hair Mask

Before you wash your hair, stir 3 tablespoons of honey and 3 tablespoons olive oil. Coat all of you hair. It is best to work in small sections. Cover hair with a plastic cap for 30 minutes. Wash and condition you hair as usual.

### Yogurt Hair Mask

Before you wash your hair, beat 1 whole egg with 1 cup of plain yogurt. Coat all of you hair. It is best to work in small sections.

Cover hair with a plastic cap for 30 minutes. Wash and condition you hair as usual.

## Egg & Olive Oil Hair Mask

After you wash your hair, beat two whole eggs with ½ cup of olive oil. Coat all of your hair. Wrap head with plastic wrap, and leave in hair for 10 minutes. Rinse well.

## Mayonnaise Conditioner for Dry Hair

Before you wash your hair, coat your hair with 1/2 cup of mayonnaise. Cover your hair with a plastic cap for 15 minutes. Rinse thoroughly. Shampoo and condition as usual.

## Hot Oil Treatment

Warm 2 to 3 tablespoons olive oil in the microwave for 15 seconds, it should not get too hot, and apply to scalp with cotton balls. Let set for 20 minutes. Shampoo and condition as usual.

## Moisturizers

Apply natural oils such as shea butter, olive oil or jojoba oil to your ends daily.

*(For best results, use raw unfiltered apple cider vinegar, found at most health food stores.)

# Conclusion

## Love Your Hair

Everything worth having takes time, patience, and a little bit of love. There are no short cuts to growing your hair. This guide is designed to help you cultivate a loving relationship with your hair so it will grow and flourish.

Having long hair is possible for all of our hair types. There are thousands of Black Women with coarse hair that has grown past their shoulders, just like there are thousands of Black women with wavy hair that doesn't seem to grow past their ears. It is not about hair type. It never was. Having long, healthy, shiny hair is about how you take care of it.

Giving your hair what it needs on a daily basis, while also avoiding damaging habits, is the only way to grow your hair. Once you learn the practice and patients for growing long hair, that practice and patience will spill over to all the areas of your life. You will learn the practice and patience to make more money, have better relationships, and most of all, have more Joy! Your life will never be the same again. This is my promise to you.

# ABOUT THE AUTHOR

*Grow Your Hair, Change Your Life* came about through my experience with growing my hair long. As a child, my sister and I had "long" hair. Our hair was longer than most black girls, although it was only to our shoulders.

My mother took care of our hair the best she knew how; washing and conditioning it every week, but also giving us tight little ponytails with elastic rubber bands that pulled hair out daily. She also added loads of grease, but we were happy with the results.

When I was twelve, she decided that I was old enough to take care of my hair myself, and with no guidance, I accepted the challenge. By the time I was 14, my hair was short, damaged and very thin. It remained that way through most of college years, where I wore braids, weaves and ponytails to hide the fact that my hair was very short. Towards my last years of college, I wore natural two-strand Twists. My hair grew fairly well, but my ends were always very dry and damaged due to the fact that I washed it only once a month. When I took the twists out, they were like little dreadlocks that I ripped through with a comb.

By the time I was in my mid-twenties, I had started wearing weaves, and wigs, to cover up a huge bald spot that just kept getting larger. I literally only had a three inch band of hair around my head and no hair in the middle.

Up until I was 26, I believed that only certain types of people, with certain types of hair, could have long hair. Then I saw my cousin, who looked just like me, with hair flowing down way past her mid-back. So my belief about who can have long hair was shattered and I began researching hair growth. I had read about growing long hair and it said that you have to cut off all of the damaged hair, so I cut my hair into a very short buzz cut and dyed it red. I created a mental picture of how long I wanted my hair and I would tell myself every time I did my hair. Once I created a loving relationship with my hair, I would notice when it was healthy and glowing or dry and under-conditioned and I could attend to it in the proper manner.

It took many years of trial and error to create all of the guidelines that I am sharing with you in this book. This book was written to help you avoid all of the mistakes I have made, and benefit from the knowledge I've learned over the years.